I0454425

NEW GUIDE TO MICRODOSING PSILOCYBIN MUSHROOMS

Psychedelic Harvest a Guide to Cultivating Well-being

Myles Albert

Copyright

All rights reserved. No part of this publication may be reproduced, distributed, or transmitted in any form or by any means, including, recording, or other electronic or mechanical methods, without the prior written permission of the publisher, except in the case of brief quotations embodied in critical reviews and certain other non-commercial uses permitted by copyright law.

© 2023 by Myles Albert

Contents

INTRODUCTION

Welcome to the "New Guide to Microdosing Psilocybin Mushrooms" where old knowledge and contemporary understanding meet. Consider this guide to be your trusty plow, breaking ground on the vast terrain of microdosing - a discipline that goes beyond horticulture to become a voyage of self-discovery.

In these pages, we're going to look into the history of psilocybin, as well as the various traditions that have sprung up around it. We'll plant the seeds of knowledge together, fostering the reasons why microdosing has emerged as a beacon of revolutionary potential in today's world.

Prepare to traverse the verdant rows of instructions on how to gently microdose in order to harvest the health and medical advantages that grow like colorful flowers in a well-tended garden. We'll answer the critical issue, "Is Microdosing right for me?" in a straightforward manner, ensuring you enter on this path with clear-eyed purpose.

Discover how to get the most out of your microdosing experience, increasing the produce of insight, creativity, and resilience as we travel through this fruitful terrain. And for those thinking of harvesting, we'll go into the art of ethically procuring psilocybin, providing a road map through the ethical and legal factors to ensure your trip is respectful.

So put on your hat, lace up your boots, and join us on this fascinating adventure. The fields of opportunity are immense, and knowledge awaits harvest. Best wishes!

Chapter 1

PSILOCYBIN AND THE EVOLUTION OF MICRODOSING

Origins and Traditions of Sowing Seeds

Consider going back to the earliest human settlements, when our forefathers discovered the enigmatic effects of psilocybin-containing mushrooms. For centuries, native tribes around the world, from the Mazatecs in Mexico to indigenous groups in Africa, have had a close relationship with these fungi.

These tribes, shrouded in ceremonial practices, incorporated Psilocybin into their rituals, viewing the mushrooms as a portal to the spiritual realm. Psilocybin mushrooms, for example, were used in healing ceremonies by the Mazatec, who believed in their ability to connect the individual with the divine.

Psilocybin mushrooms continued to weave into many cultural traditions as time unfolded its tapestry. The work of researchers like Albert Hofmann and Timothy Leary increased the attention of Western civilizations to these fungi in the twentieth century. Their research and experiences opened the way for a better knowledge of psilocybin and helped pave the way for the modern phenomenon of microdosing.

Developing Curiosity: New Insights into Psilocybin

We are now in the twenty-first century, a time of scientific study and rediscovery. Researchers, curious minds, and activists have sifted through the stigma to uncover Psilocybin's potential advantages, including its ability to favorably affect mental health.

Psilocybin's neurological effects have been studied in depth, giving insight into its interaction with serotonin receptors in the brain. Once dismissed as a simple delusion, the psychedelic experience is today acknowledged as a complex interaction of neurotransmitters that may have therapeutic effects.

Furthermore, the renewed interest in microdosing Psilocybin has sparked a new wave of study. The study of the subtle effects of taking modest, regular dosages of psilocybin is now underway, with encouraging results in terms of understanding its impact on mood, cognition, and overall well-being.

As we go through the history of psilocybin and microdosing, we find ourselves at a crossroads of tradition and innovation. Knowledge has deep roots, and seeds of inquiry continue to blossom, allowing us to explore the enormous breadth of this ancient yet ever-evolving activity.

Chapter 2

REASONS FOR MICRODOSING PSILOCYBIN

Mental and Emotional Well-Being

Mind Nourishment

Microdosing, which is similar to gently watering a garden, has been linked to improved mental health. Psilocybin, the active component, is like nutrient-rich rain that feeds the mind. According to research, microdosing may help with mood improvement and the relief of symptoms associated with sadness and anxiety.

Scientific research has grown up to investigate the effects of psilocybin on the brain. According to these findings, microdosing may increase serotonin receptors, the soil in which happy moods commonly grow.

Personal Gardens: Many people have shared their personal tales, noting that microdosing was like sunlight bursting through the clouds on a rainy day. There have been reports of improved mood, greater emotions of joy, and an overall sense of well-being.

Remove the Unwanted: Anxiety and Depression

Consider your mind to be a garden, and worry and despair to be troublesome weeds. Some feel that microdosing can act as a natural herbicide, assisting in the management of these unwelcome

16

visitors. According to some studies, the effects of microdosing may help to quiet the hyperactive areas of the brain linked with anxiety and sadness.

Case Studies: People who have incorporated microdosing into their lives have experienced reduced anxiety and removed clouds of despair. It's like plucking out the invasive weeds to allow the flowers to blossom.

However, it is critical to explore these sectors with caution. While some people feel alleviation, others may experience increased worry or pain. Like in any garden, what works for one plant may not work for another.

Increasing Resilience Through Creativity and Problem Solving

Developing Creativity

Consider your mind to be a large landscape, with creativity acting as the wildflowers that color it. Some mental gardeners feel that microdosing functions as a specific fertilizer, increasing creativity and improving the way people think.

Sprouting Ideas: Some users have observed that microdosing allows them to perceive things in a new light. It's like caring for your mental garden and uncovering fresh, brilliant flowers of ideas.

Artists, authors, and musicians have related stories on how microdosing has affected their creative processes. It's like a spark that ignites the fire of creativity, allowing you to create masterpieces on the canvas of your mind.

Working Through Issues

Life's challenges are like boulders in the soil—unavoidable yet controllable. Some say that microdosing, like a competent plow, makes traversing hurdles and problem solving easier.

Fertile Solutions: Microdosers claim to be more adaptive when faced with problems. It's as if the mental soil gets more fertile, allowing problem-solving seeds to germinate and develop.

Harvest of Insight: Users have described receiving fresh views on old concerns as if microdosing is a type of mental tilling, unearthing buried insights ready to blossom.

Wrapping it up

The reasons for microdosing psilocybin mushrooms are as varied as the crops grown on a well-tended farm. Microdosing is a gardener's toolset for the mind, with benefits ranging from mental well-being to creativity and problem-solving. However, just as different plants require different care, microdosing may not be appropriate for everyone. As we continue our exploration of this field of knowledge, we'll look at the concerns and safeguards to take before proceeding.

Chapter 3

NURTURING THE PLANT

Choosing the Right Mushrooms: Gathering the Right Seeds

First and foremost, before embarking on this adventure, you must be familiar with mushrooms. Because not every fungus in the pasture is edible, farmers must exercise caution. Psilocybin-containing mushrooms are the stars of our show, and typical cultivars include Psilocybe cubensis, Psilocybe semilanceata, and Psilocybe mexicana.

Make certain you can recognize these guys. Consult field guides, internet information, or an experienced picker. Remember, we don't want any wild mushrooms wreaking havoc like a fox in the henhouse.

You may now obtain these magical mushrooms in two ways: cultivate them yourself or trade seeds with someone who has a green thumb.

How to Grow Your Own Mushrooms

Consider raising your own pilocybin mushrooms to be similar to caring for a vegetable garden. You'll need the following items:

Spawn or Spores

Begin with spores or spawn—it's similar to sowing seeds. These are available online or from knowledgeable growers. They're the heart and soul of your mushroom business.

Support

The substrate—the soil for your mushrooms—will be required next. Brown rice flour, vermiculite, and water should be combined. It's similar to preparing the ideal atmosphere for your seeds to develop.

Packaging

Consider containers as the pots for your mushrooms. Allow them to develop and thrive in jars or bags. spot them in a warm, dark spot and watch your sprouts grow.

Air that is both light and fresh

When your mushrooms begin to emerge, expose them to light and fresh air. It's similar to allowing the sun and air to strike your plants— they adore it.

Gathering

Harvest your mushrooms when they are mature and ready, just like you would ripe tomatoes. Gently twist them, and you've got yourself a homemade harvest.

Remember that patience is essential. It's similar to seeing corn grow—you can't hurry it.

Ethical and Legal Considerations in Seed Trading

If gardening isn't your thing or you want a quick fix, you may now swap seeds with those who have already planted. But before you start haggling like it's a county fair, there are a few things to consider.

Ethical Trading Practices

Make sure your deals are fair and square, just as you wouldn't trade a donkey for a sack of beans. Be truthful, and treat others as you would like to be treated. It's the golden rule of both farming and trade.

Legal Limits

Let us now discuss the legal structure of the land. Psilocybin mushrooms are still as illegal in many locations as a fox in a cabbage patch. Make sure you are familiar with the legislation in your region. Keep everything lawful and low-key; we don't want any run-ins with the sheriff.

Now that you've obtained the mushrooms, let's go on to the next stage of our microdosing saga.

Field Maintenance: Dosage and Frequency

Consider dosing to be similar to feeding your crops; you want exactly the correct amount—not too much or too little. If you use too little, you won't see much development; use too much, and you can wind yourself up with a bunch of problems. Let's dissect it.

Determining the Appropriate Dosage

Begin slowly and steadily, as if you were sowing seeds in a furrow. A typical psilocybin microdose ranges from 0.1 to 0.5 grams—just enough to give your mental crops a mild boost without throwing them into a psychedelic frenzy.

Consider your physical weight as well as your tolerance. It's similar to fertilizing your garden according to the size of your plot. A smaller garden requires less fertilizer, and a lighter body may require a lower amount.

Exploring the Frequency

Let's speak about how frequently you should water your crops now. Microdosing is analogous to irrigating your thoughts on a regular, but not excessive, basis. Begin with a timetable, such as every third day. It's similar to watching the weather: you want to give your plants adequate water but don't want them to drown.

Keep a journal—perhaps name it your "Harvest Log"—and record your experiences. Take note of the dosage, the effects, and how it affects your daily life. It's similar to keeping track of weather patterns— it helps you forecast when the sun will shine and when it will rain.

Harvesting the Bounty: Microdosing in Everyday Life

After you've planted your seeds and cared for your crops, it's time to reap your rewards and put those mushrooms to good use. Putting microdosing into your everyday life is similar to putting fresh vegetables into your meals—it provides a little something extra without taking up the entire plate.

Morning Routines

Consider giving your crops the first rays of sunshine by taking your microdose in the morning. It creates a good tone for the day, preparing you to tackle whatever problems may arise.

Mindfulness Exercises

Consider microdosing as a tool to help you improve your mindful practices, whether they be meditation, yoga, or simply taking a leisurely stroll through the fields. It's like lovingly and attentively tending to your crops.

Reflection and Modification

Maintain vigilance on your harvest log. Adjust your dosage or frequency if you see any problems, such as undesired side effects or disturbances. It's similar to plucking out invasive plants that are threatening your crop.

Remember that microdosing is a process, not a race. Take your time, observe, and make adjustments as necessary. It's like seeing the seasons change—each stage has a role in the vast cycle of development.

Chapter 4

MICRODOSING'S HEALTH AND MEDICAL BENEFITS

Potential Therapeutic Benefits

Microdosing is similar to caring for a plant's roots; it may not be spectacular, but it is where the true magic occurs. Many people feel that psilocybin microdosing might work as a natural fertilizer for the mind and body, stimulating development and vitality. Let's have a look at some of the possible therapeutic outcomes.

Mind Nourishment

The fascinating component present in these mushrooms, psilocybin, has been shown to interact with serotonin receptors in the brain. Serotonin, sometimes known as the "feel-good" neurotransmitter, is important in mood regulation. Some microdosers report an increase in mood, anxiety reduction, and general mental well-being.

It's like pouring a soft rain on your thoughts—not too much to flood the fields, but just enough to grow the seeds of optimism.

Developing Creativity

Consider your mind to be a large field waiting to be sown with seeds of invention. Some microdosers suggest that a daily dosage of psilocybin may boost creativity. The mind becomes a fertile place for creation when ideas flourish like wildflowers. Breakthroughs and new perspectives on creative efforts have been reported by artists, authors, and intellectuals.

The mushrooms act as a natural fertilizer, strengthening the soil of your mind so that creativity may develop and bloom.

Trauma and PTSD Care

Trauma may be like a persistent weed in the mind's garden, impeding development and creating anguish.

According to certain research, microdosing psilocybin may have therapeutic benefits for those suffering from post-traumatic stress disorder (PTSD). Psilocybin's soft touch may help remove the hold of unpleasant memories, enabling healing to take root.

Consider it a soft wind that helps to take away the debris of previous storms, leaving behind a more calm scene.

Planting Mindfulness Seeds

The mind, like a neglected garden overtaken by weeds, may get crowded in the hurry and bustle of contemporary life. Psilocybin microdosing has been linked to improved awareness and a stronger connection to the present moment. It's like a gardener's touch, caring for the garden of the mind with care, ensuring that each moment is enjoyed and relished.

Tilling the Safety Soil

Before you begin the journey of microdosing, you must first assess your mental health background. Certain situations, like any agricultural enterprise, may not be favorable to growing certain crops. Individuals who have a personal or familial history of psychotic illnesses should exercise caution, since psilocybin may worsen such problems.

Before going into the realm of microdosing, always check with a mental health specialist. It's similar to having a seasoned farmer inspect your soil before you plant your seeds to ensure the conditions are ideal for a good yield.

Misuse and Dependence Weeds

While the intricacy of microdosing is frequently commended, it is critical to resist the temptation of overindulgence. Microdosing isn't a call to a psychedelic party in your head; it's more like a constant drizzle than a thunderstorm. Regular, regulated dosages are essential; excessive usage may result in dependency or undesirable side effects.

Consider it like watering your plants: too much and they will drown; too little and they will wither. A successful garden requires consistency.

Legal Terrain Navigation

There are legal issues when it comes to psilocybin, just as there are restrictions concerning what you can and cannot grow in your garden. The laws governing these miraculous mushrooms vary greatly, and it is important to be informed of the legal situation in your area.

It's similar to knowing local regulations; you wouldn't want to cultivate a prohibited crop and risk attracting the wrath of the authorities. Before you plant your seeds, learn the lay of the land.

Potential Side Effects of Weathering

Every garden has storms, and microdosing is no exception. While most people report favorable results, others may have adverse effects such as nausea, anxiety, or changes in perception. It's critical to be prepared for these possible storms and approach microdosing with a resilient mentality.

Consider it like being prepared for inclement weather, such as bringing an umbrella in case of rain or sunscreen in case of sun. Preparedness facilitates an easier

ride   through   the   microdosing
seasons.

Chapter 5

EXAMINING THE SITUATION: IS MICRODOSING RIGHT FOR ME?

Considerations and Precautions When Plowing Through Weeds

Before you go fully into the realm of microdosing, there are a few things you should know. You must be aware of your mental and physical terrain, just as you would check the weather before sowing seeds. Here are a few things to think about:

Know Your Soil: Mental Health Evaluation

Consider your mind to be soil, and before you plant any seeds, you want to know whether it's fruitful ground. It's like planting on rough soil if you're coping with major mental health difficulties. Microdosing may not be the right crop for you. It is critical to consult with a mental health specialist, just as it is to talk with an experienced farmer. They will assist you in determining if your soil is ready for the seeds.

Medications and Interactions for Weed Control

Some drugs and psilocybin do not mix well, much as some plants do not get along in the same patch. It's a good idea to see your doctor if you're using any prescription medications. When you combine them, they may inform you whether any unfavorable weeds will sprout. Always put safety first.

Crop Rotation: Trauma and Past Experiences

Bad plants from the past might sometimes be found in the soil. Trauma and difficult events may be like tenacious plants that must be removed. It's important to be aware that microdosing may cause emotional turmoil. It's similar to making sure your grounds are ready before planting.

Setting and Environment

Your surroundings are important, just as certain plants like sunshine while others prefer shade. Microdosing is not something to be taken lightly. You must choose the appropriate time and location, such as sowing seeds while the sun is shining. Choose a location that makes you feel secure and at ease. It's important to provide the ideal circumstances for your seeds to thrive.

Microdosing Personal Reflections

Let's speak about you, the farmer, caring for this mental garden now that we've examined the soil. It is important to reflect on your own ideas and emotions. It's similar to designing your garden layout—

where to plant what and how much room each crop needs.

What Do You Want to Grow?

Consider what you want to gain from microdosing. Do you want to improve your creativity, get rid of worry, or simply feel better in general? It's like picking your crops correctly; each one has its own set of advantages. Setting specific objectives is similar to sowing seeds with a purpose.

Expectations and Goals

Set reasonable objectives for your microdosing journey, just as you would for your garden rows. Perhaps you want to improve your attention at work or discover more pleasure in your daily life. Recognize that microdosing is not a quick remedy but rather like sowing seeds and seeing them develop over time. Patience is the fertilizer that allows your dreams to sprout.

Start with a small patch of soil

Begin microdosing with a modest amount, just as you would when evaluating the soil before a large planting. The field is your thoughts, and it's always best to be careful at the beginning. A little patch allows you to examine how the soil responds without affecting the rest of the garden.

Schedule for Watering— Dosage and Frequency

Dosage and frequency are important considerations in microdosing, just as they are when selecting how often to water your plants. It's all about striking the correct balance between too much and too little. Just as plants need continuous watering, your mind requires a steady supply of the appropriate quantity of psilocybin.

Support System for Companion Plants

Consider your surroundings and your support system. Having others who understand and support your path is critical, just as some plants help each other thrive. Talking to friends or joining groups of like-minded people might be compared to having companion plants in your yard.

Chapter 6

MAKING THE MOST OF MICRODOSING

Mindfulness and Conscious Living

1. <u>The Mindfulness Seed</u>

Microdosing is more than merely popping a mushroom and going about your business like a scarecrow in the field. It is about sowing the seed of awareness—being aware and present in the present moment. Consider it like watering your mental garden.

2. Developing the Habit

Mindfulness isn't a one-time event; it's a steady rainfall. Pay attention to your thoughts, emotions, and sensations while microdosing. Take note of how the rain of awareness feeds your thoughts. Be a skillful farmer, carefully caring for each sprout.

3. Eliminate distractions

Distractions are like bothersome weeds in your harvest in today's environment. Mindfulness assists you in identifying and extracting them. When microdosing, aim to keep the area devoid of extraneous noise and disruptions. Allow your mind to be the tranquil paradise it was designed to be.

Setting and Achieving Goals in the Light of Intention

1. Planting intentional seeds

Set specific aims for your microdosing journey, just as you would when determining what crops to cultivate. What do you hope to accomplish? Be explicit about your goals, whether they are to increase creativity, reduce anxiety, or acquire clarity. Your intentions are the seeds that will grow into the consequences you want.

2. Maintain your garden on a regular basis

Goals, like plants, need frequent attention. Check in with your intentions on a frequent basis. Is your watering schedule correct, or do you need to make changes? Maybe your ambitions have increased, and it's time to shine some light on them. Regular introspection ensures that your garden remains healthy and bright.

3. Reaping the Benefits of Your Labor

Celebrate your accomplishments when the time comes to harvest what you've planted. Have you seen a boost in productivity or a fresh feeling of calm? Recognize and cherish the good improvements microdosing brings to your life, just as a farmer loves the crop.

In simple terms, extensive detail

1. Microdosing with Mindfulness

Consider mindfulness to be like nurturing your mental garden. Just as plants need water to bloom, your mind requires awareness to thrive. When you're attentive, you're paying attention to what's going on in the present. It's like sitting in the rain while caring for your crops.

Mindfulness is a practice in microdosing. It is not a torrential rain that floods your fields; rather, it is a continuous drizzle that feeds every idea, emotion, and experience. Consider sitting in the garden and watching your mental flora flourish. That is what it means to be aware when microdosing.

2. Eliminating distractions

Consider distractions to be tenacious weeds that threaten to suck the life out of your crops. When you're microdosing, having a distraction-free atmosphere is akin to removing these bothersome invaders from your mental garden.

Turning off unneeded sounds is like plucking weeds. Find a peaceful place to let your thoughts rest. Mindfulness and microdosing complement each other; while you're present and attentive, your mental garden thrives.

3. Setting Goals: Planting the Seeds

Setting intentions is analogous to selecting which crops to sow. You wouldn't just spread seeds and hope for the best, would you? Similarly, when it comes to microdosing, be explicit about your goals. Are you wanting to decrease stress, increase creativity, or gain mental clarity?

Intentions are mental seeds that you plant. They direct the development of your microdosing experience. You determine what results you desire from your microdosing journey, just like a farmer chooses which crops to harvest.

4. <u>Regular Care for Your Mental Garden</u>

Your mental garden, like any other, requires frequent care. Check in with your intentions on a frequent basis. It's similar to wandering around your fields to observe how your crops are doing. Do they receive enough sunlight? Is there evidence of stress or overgrowth?

This frequent check-in assures that you're on track. Adjust your care regimen if your objectives have changed. Just like a farmer understands when to water more or add nutrients, you'll adjust your microdosing practices to meet your changing demands.

5. Celebrating Success

Celebrate your victories when it's time to harvest. Did you notice an increase in attention, a decrease in anxiety, or an increase in creativity? Recognize and relish the wonderful changes that microdosing provides, just as a farmer appreciates the wealth of the field.

Harvest is a time for introspection and joy. Your objectives have manifested into actual results. Enjoy the results of your effort, and keep in mind that, just as a farmer prepares for the following season, you may set new goals for your continuous microdosing adventure.

Chapter 7

HARVESTING WISDOM

Growing Your Own

Mushrooms

Growing your own mushrooms may be a truly satisfying effort if you want to be a genuine farmer of your own psychedelic patch. To get you started, here's a step-by-step guide:

Obtaining the Required Equipment

First and foremost, you will need the appropriate tools for the work.

Take a look at:

Vermiculite, brown rice flour, and water are used as the substrate.

Spores are the mystical seeds of your psychedelic adventure.

Containers for growing: Trays or jars for your substrate and spores.

Misting bottle: Use this to keep your growth environment moist.

Growing medium: a location for your mushrooms to live, such as a grow bag or jars.

Sowing the Seeds

Make the substrate: Combine the vermiculite, brown rice flour, and water until the mixture is wet and crumbly. Fill your growing containers with it.

Spore Inoculation: Using a syringe, inject your spores into the substrate. Consider it similar to putting little seeds in a hallucinogenic garden.

Incubate: Put your containers in a warm place and leave them in the dark for a few weeks. This is similar to the germination stage of your miraculous harvest.

Introduce Light: When you see white mycelium strands, it's time to bring in some light. This represents the light breaking through the clouds to find your mushroom blooms.

Wait for Harvest: Be patient, just as you would wait for tomatoes to mature on the vine. It's time to harvest your mushrooms once their caps appear.

Reaping the Benefits of Your Labor

Snip those mushrooms at the base, just above the substrate, using a clean knife or scissors.

Remove any remaining fragments to keep your growing place neat.

Dry them out: To dry your crop, use a food dehydrator or a low-temperature oven. Store them in an airtight container, just as you would a jar of pickles.

Learning from Errors

Farmers understand that not every season yields a bountiful harvest. Contamination, poor development, and unexpected guests (not the nice type) are all possibilities. Learn from each harvest, tweak your techniques, and keep growing.

Trading Seeds: Ethical and Legal Issues

Let us now discuss trading—not in the market sense, but in the sense of obtaining psilocybin from others. It is critical to traverse this terrain with caution, keeping both ethical and legal bounds in mind.

Trading Ethics

Community Bonds: Meet other people who are passionate about using psychedelics responsibly and respectfully. Such relationships might be made via online forums, local meet-ups, or community activities.

Transparent Dealings: Be clear and honest about your goals while negotiating with someone. The soil in which ethical trade flourishes is trust.

Pay It Forward: Consider the age-old practice of reciprocity. If someone assists you, consider how you may contribute to the well-being of others in exchange.

Getting Through the Legal Maze

Know Your Local Laws: Just as you wouldn't plant tomatoes in places where they won't grow, don't participate in actions that might put you in hot water. Investigate and comprehend the legal status of psilocybin in your location.

Personal Use vs. Distribution: Understand the legal ramifications of your aim. It's one thing if you're collecting for personal use. If you're distributing, proceed with caution since the legal repercussions might differ.

Risk and Responsibility: Be aware of the dangers involved and accept responsibility for your decisions. Laws, like the seasons, may change, so remain up-to-date.

Recognizing Trustworthy Sources

If you aren't ready to cultivate your own or trade isn't your thing, you may try traversing the jungle of available supplies. To separate the mushrooms from the toadstools, do the following:

Trustworthy Vendors

Look for providers with a proven track record. Read reviews, ask around, and be sure they're dedicated to quality and safety.

Transparency: Reputable sellers are upfront about their goods, from the origin of their spores to the growing environment.

Customer service: A good vendor is similar to a trustworthy neighbor. They are there to answer your questions, resolve your issues, and ensure that you have a pleasant experience.

Quality Control

Testing and analysis: Reputable providers test their goods for purity and efficacy. This is analogous to a farmer inspecting the soil for quality and nutrients before planting.

Consistency is important. Trustworthy suppliers aim for consistency in their goods. Look for consistency in your psilocybin, just like you would in a batch of apples.

User Feedback: Pay attention to what others have to say. If a single source continually produces a substandard crop, it's time to look for better pastures.

Privacy and Security

Discreet packing: A respectable provider recognizes the need for discrete packing. Your privacy is just as valuable as a farmer's secret recipe.

Secure Payment Methods: Make certain that your transactions are safe. Reliable suppliers provide secure and discrete payment alternatives to safeguard both parties.

CONCLUSION

We've sowed the seeds of knowledge in the lush fields of microdosing, nurtured the delicate shoots of insight, and gathered the wisdom that emerges from responsible research. As we get to the end of "The Complete Guide to Microdosing Psilocybin," imagine your mind as a growing garden, nourished by the complex sensations and insights revealed. Whether you choose to grow your own mushrooms, trade with other mushroom hunters, or buy from reputable sellers, keep in mind that the harvest is a personal experience. Approach it with respect, accountability, and an open heart. The landscape of your awareness awaits, ready to bloom with the brilliant hues of well-being and wisdom. Happy harvesting, and may your microdosing adventures bring you a feast of blossoming moments and fresh insight.